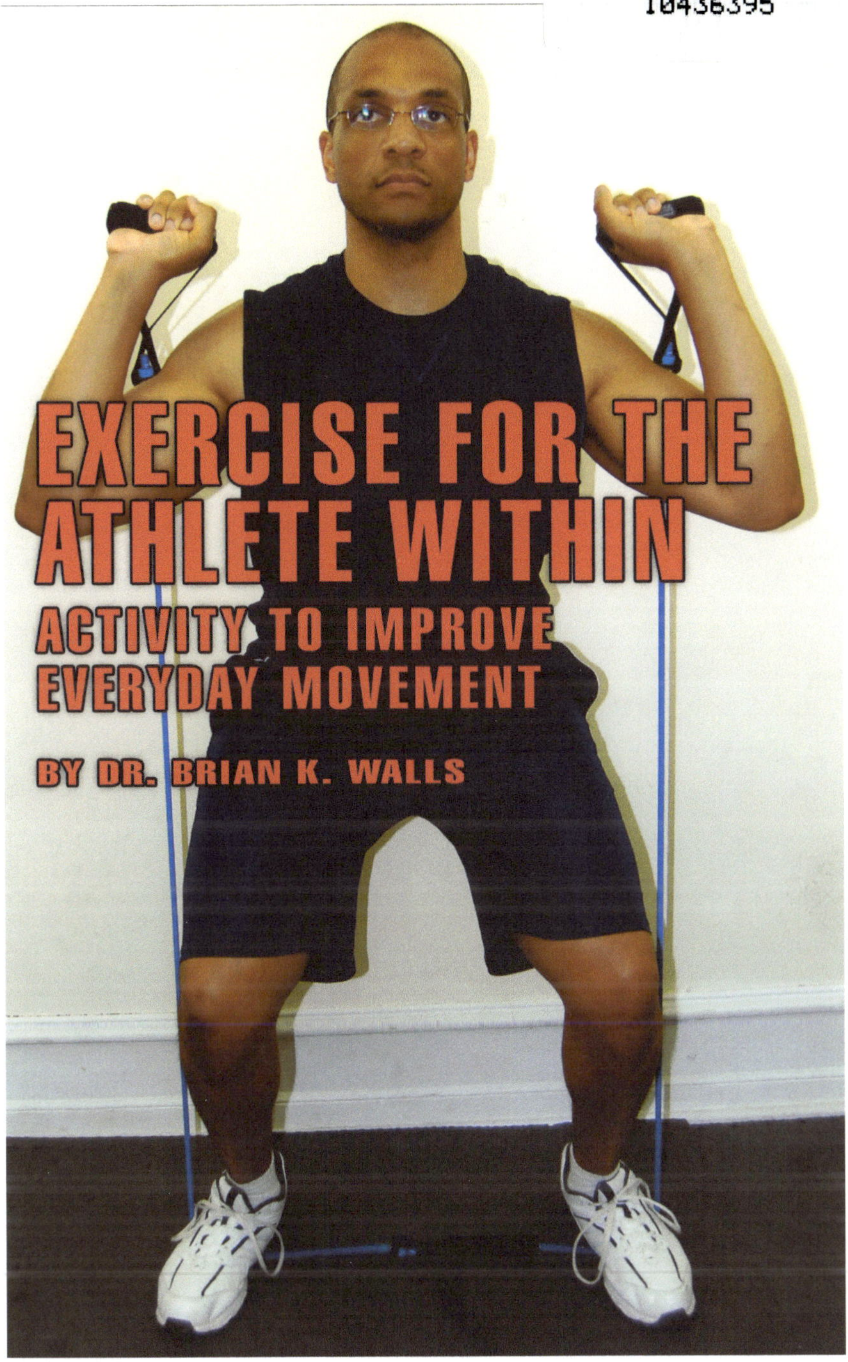

EXERCISE FOR THE ATHLETE WITHIN
ACTIVITY TO IMPROVE EVERYDAY MOVEMENT

BY DR. BRIAN K. WALLS

Dr. Brian K. Walls

ISBN:1478398892
ISBN-13:9781478398899

CONTENTS

DEDICATION

DEDICATED TO MY BEST FRIEND AND TEAMMATE FOR LIFE.
MY LOVING WIFE

ACKNOWLEDGMENTS

A special thank you goes to Dennis James, Barry James and Troy Hendricks, the guys who helped to make this book possible.

FORWARD

HUMAN BEINGS WERE MADE TO MOVE

When we're young, we could not wait to move about our environment. Take a moment and remember the childlike rush of excitement when we were told that it was time for recess. We are built to walk, jump and run. However, for the most part, people in the 21st century have decided that moving just does not fit into their daily schedules. All of us create reasons not to move: I do not have enough time to exercise, I am too tired to exercise, or I have too much to do to exercise. Does this sound familiar? I do not want anyone to be misguided into thinking that I have not said these things to myself as well! Moving allows our muscles to pump blood throughout the body. Moving helps decrease the stress of the day. Moving, regardless of the activity, makes us feel good.

So as you, the reader, pick up this book, take a moment and recall the feelings of excitement when you were all allowed to go outside and play. Think of this book as a beginners manual on how to make your body move for a few minutes a day.

CONTACT YOUR PHYSICIAN BEFORE EXERCISING

Exercise is not without risk. To reduce the risk of injury, please consult with your physician for safety precautions and appropriate exercise prescription. Also, never forget that if you are experiencing any pain, STOP performing the exercise and consult your physician. Have fun!

MOVEMENT 1: THE ART OF BREATHING

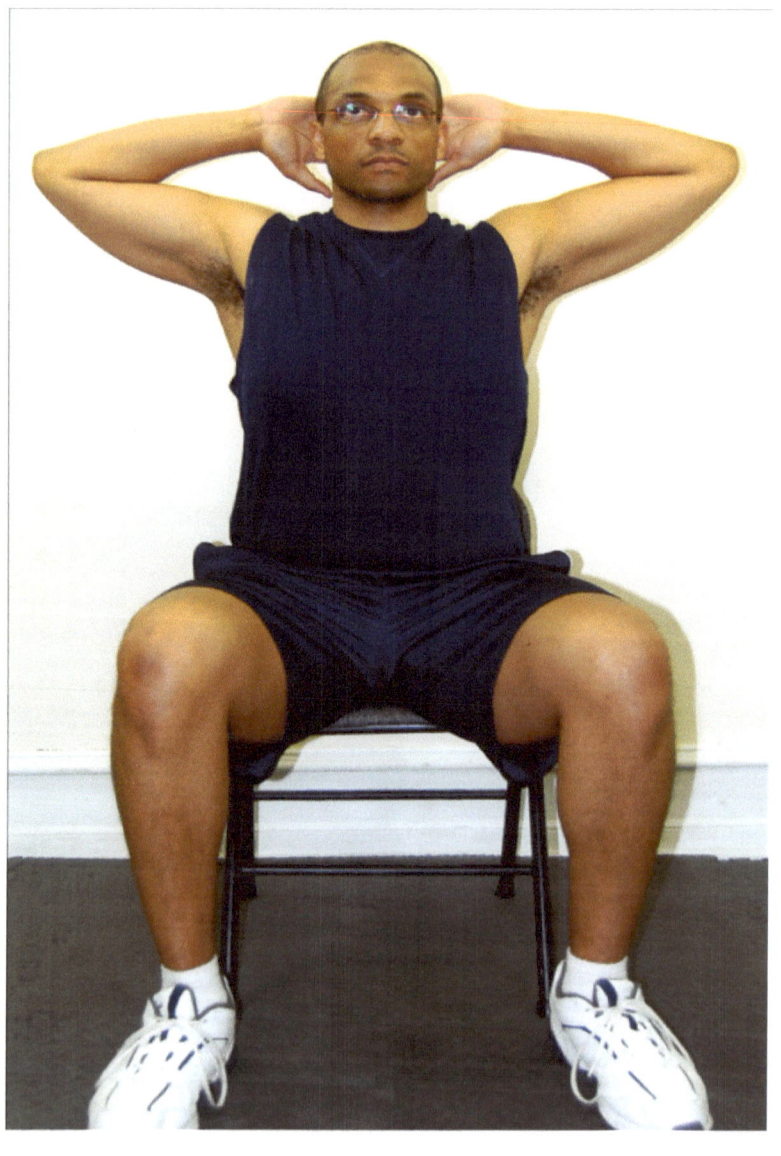

ARE YOU BREATHING EFFECTIVELY?

If you're reading this page, you're undoubtedly breathing. That being said, the question remains, are you breathing as effectively as you should be? The answer is probably a resounding NO. Right now you are thinking that I am crazy and for the most part, you're probably correct. However, take a moment and concentrate on your breathing. Do your shoulders rise when you take a breath? Does your stomach become larger, as if your stomach was a balloon? Do you breathe in through your mouth and out through your nose? Before you continue reading, sit back and just breathe for one minute.

What did you notice? Did your shoulders move up in a classic 'I don't know' position? Did your chest move farther than your stomach? Did your stomach move farther than your chest?

I am sure that these questions as well as a number of other questions, came to your mind, which is exactly what should happen! As humans, we take breathing for granted. The only time in our lives that we are concerned about our breathing is when we stop breathing. Think about that for a moment...we are only concerned about breathing when we're NOT breathing. That is a very morbid way of thinking about breathing.

So the question arises, why is breathing so important?

First of all, breathing is what keeps us alive. Well no duh! You do not need me to tell you that. Second, breathing brings oxygen to our cells, which will create energy for our body. I think we all can use a little more energy in our daily lives! Third, by breathing from our stomach, or diaphragm, we utilize our primary breathing muscles. This action relaxes the muscles around the neck and shoulders, otherwise known as our secondary breathing muscles. The end result bring that by learning proper breathing techniques, you will decrease the overall stress on the muscles of your body.

Now that you understand what proper breathing means to you, it is time to work on improving our breathing!

When performing these breathing exercises, make sure that you are seated in a quiet room and that you give yourself 2 minutes a day to perform the exercises. You read that correctly! 2 minutes a day is all I am asking of you. I am optimistic that you can spare 2 minutes in your busy schedule for yourself. There are two breathing exercises that everyone should perform to improve their breathing. The first exercise is called Helpful Hands. The Helpful Hands exercise will show you how you breathe. Once again, that may sound a little strange to you, but most of us do not know how we breathe.

Here is how you perform the Helpful Hands exercise:

1. Sit down in a comfortable chair, with your back supported, shoulders back and your feet shoulder width apart and flat on the ground.
2. Take your dominant hand (the hand that you write with) and place it on your chest.
3. Take your other hand and place it on your stomach.
4. Now take 3 breaths. The hand that moves the farthest will indicate if you are a shallow breather (someone who breathes from their chest), or a deep breather (someone who breathes from their diaphragm).

Shallow Breather

A shallow breather is someone who breathes from their chest, which is not the optimal breathing pattern. Shallow breathers use their neck and shoulder muscles, or secondary muscles, to inflate the lungs. This type of breathing leads to overworked, or stressed, secondary muscles; muscles that normally hold a great deal of our everyday stresses. So we should try to decrease the stress we place on our secondary muscles!

Deep Breather

A deep breather is someone who breathes from their stomach, or diaphragm, which is the optimal breathing pattern. Deep breathers use their diaphragm, a muscle at the base of our lungs, to inflate the lungs. This type of breathing leads to a natural breathing pattern which relaxes our secondary muscles.

Once you have determined the type of breather you are, you are now ready to move on to the next exercise which is called the Balloon. This exercise will help you to become a better overall breather by utilizing your entire lung capacity.

Here is how you perform the Balloon exercise:

1. Sit down in a comfortable chair, with your back supported, shoulders back and your feet shoulder width apart and flat on the ground. You may also perform this exercise while lying down in your bed, flat on your back.
2. Take both hands and place them on your stomach, with your fingers interlocked.
3. Close your eyes and breathe in through your nose and then out through your   mouth. With each breath you should be "blowing" up your internal Balloon (your stomach), so that your fingers separate from one another on each inhalation and come together on each exhalation.
4. Perform 10 deep breaths.
5. **WARNING:** You may fall asleep while performing this exercise! DO NOT perform this exercise while using heavy machinery.

Both of the aforementioned exercises will relax you as well as help you breathe better. By incorporating the Art of Breathing, you are using your entire lung capacity by filling up your lungs and body with its full complement of oxygen. The exercises may be extended for longer periods of time, but start off with 2 minutes so that you may become accustomed to the exercise and the feeling of improved breathing. In the beginning, you may want to set an alarm clock so that you do not oversleep. Enjoy breathing!

MOVEMENT 2: STRETCHES TO KEEP YOU FLEXIBLE

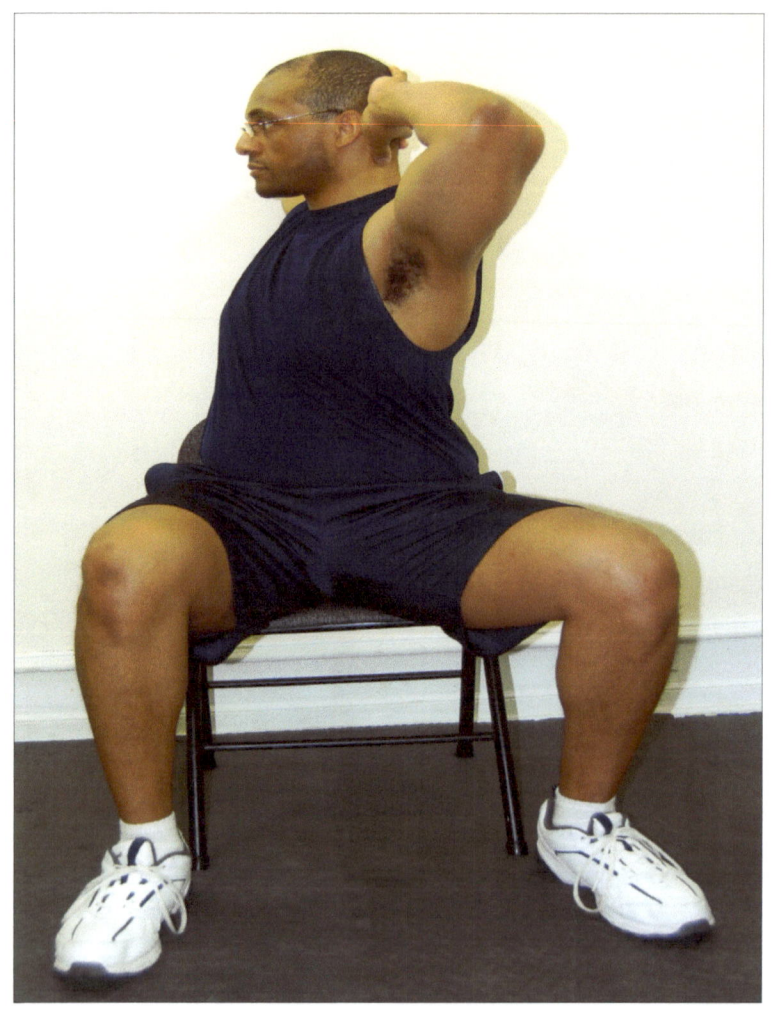

The Human Body is perhaps one of the most amazing and well made pieces of machinery that has ever been created. If I may stand up on my pulpit for a moment, the great scientist that created us knew what he or she was doing! With that being said, it is a wonder how little we take care of our own bodies. Perhaps the simplest way to help ourselves is to stretch every day.

Before you sit back and think that I am asking you to perform something crazy and out of the ordinary, take a look at your pet or an animal after it wakes from a nap. What is the first thing that it does? The animal stretches! Have you ever heard of an animal complaining about a tight muscle? I will wager that while reading this paragraph you just complained about some part of your body being tight. Humans are one of the few animals that do not stretch after waking from hours of slumber, but still think that we should be able to move without pain or discomfort. Before we move on to the stretches that will keep you moving, let me run down a normal day for most people:

Wake up, get out of bed, go to the bathroom, brush your teeth, shower, get dressed, eat ("grab") breakfast and go to a car, bus or train (where we sit!) to a career that we…. (You guessed it!) go and sit. Sound familiar? The order of the day may change, but the premise is still the same. We are all moving around on tight muscles that may lead to aches and pains that could be avoided by just taking 3 minutes a day to stretch. Does not sound so bad when you realize that all you have to do is 3 minutes, 180 seconds a day and you may be able to help yourself move better. I have to make this statement, or my lawyer will be very upset with me. Please consult your physician before performing any of the stretches or exercises. If you experience any discomfort or pain, **stop** the stretch or exercise and consult your physician. Without further ado, here are the stretches that will keep you moving!

STRAIGHT LEG STRETCH

This is a simple stretch that can be performed in bed either the moment after you wake up and before you go to bed. You can also perform this exercise while at work at your desk. Remember all you need is 3 minutes a day; 60 seconds in the morning, afternoon and night! This stretch helps to stretch the muscles of the back of the legs. Here is how the Straight Leg Stretch is performed:

1. Start in a seated position, keep your legs straight in front of you and your toes pointed toward the ceiling with heels on the bed/floor.
2. Without bending your knees, reach for your toes. Stop stretching once you feel a slight stretch in the back of your legs.
3. Hold this stretch for 10 seconds. Do not worry if you cannot reach your toes… Rome was not built in one day!

TWIST STRETCH

This is a stretch that you should perform following the Straight Leg Stretch. This stretch is for the lower back muscles and can also be performed in bed or while at work. Here is how the Twist Stretch is performed:

1. Start in a seated position, keep your legs straight in front of you and your toes pointed toward the ceiling with heels on the bed/floor.
2. Without bending your knees, look over your right shoulder by turning your torso, at the waist, to the right. **Hold** this position for 10 seconds.
3. After 10 seconds, return to the start position.
4. **Slowly** turn your head looking over your left shoulder, turning your torso, at the waist, to the left. **Hold** this position for 10 seconds.

CAMEL BACK STRETCH

This stretch focuses on stretching the upper back muscles that may become tight due to the countless hours that you may spend in your car or at your computer. Here is how the Camel Back Stretch is performed:

1. Start in a seated position, with your legs straight in front of you and with your toes pointed toward the ceiling with heels on the bed/floor.
2. Extend your arms and bring both hands in front of you and raise your arms to chest level.
3. Close your hands together, bring your chin to your chest and **slowly** reach in front of you rounding out your back
4. Hold this position for 10 seconds.

EAR TO SHOULDER STRETCH

This stretch focuses on stretching out the muscles on the side of your neck. You know, those muscles that you are always stretching while working at the computer or in your car sitting in traffic. Here is how the Ear to Shoulder Stretch is performed:

1. Start in a seated position, with your legs straight in front of you and your toes pointed toward the ceiling with your heels on the bed/floor. Place your arms on the side of your body.
2. Relax your shoulders and bend your right ear towards your shoulder. Hold your position the moment you feel a slight stretch at your left shoulder.
3. Hold the stretch for 10 seconds.
4. After 10 seconds, **slowly** bend your left ear to your left shoulder. Hold your position the moment you feel a slight stretch at your right shoulder.
5. Hold the stretch for 10 seconds

Congratulations! You have just completed the Stretches that will keep you moving. Great job! Can you believe that all it took was 60 seconds? Of course, if you have more time, you can repeat any stretch or do the entire routine again.

HOW TO CHOOSE THE CORRECT RESISTANCE BAND/TUBE

Choosing the correct resistance band/tube can be difficult without prior knowledge of the resistance classifications. Below is a quick and easy classification list of the resistance of the band/tubes.

COLOR	LEVEL
Yellow	Extra Light
Red	Medium
Blue	Heavy
Purple	Extra Heavy

MOVEMENT 3: EXERCISES TO KEEP YOU STRONG

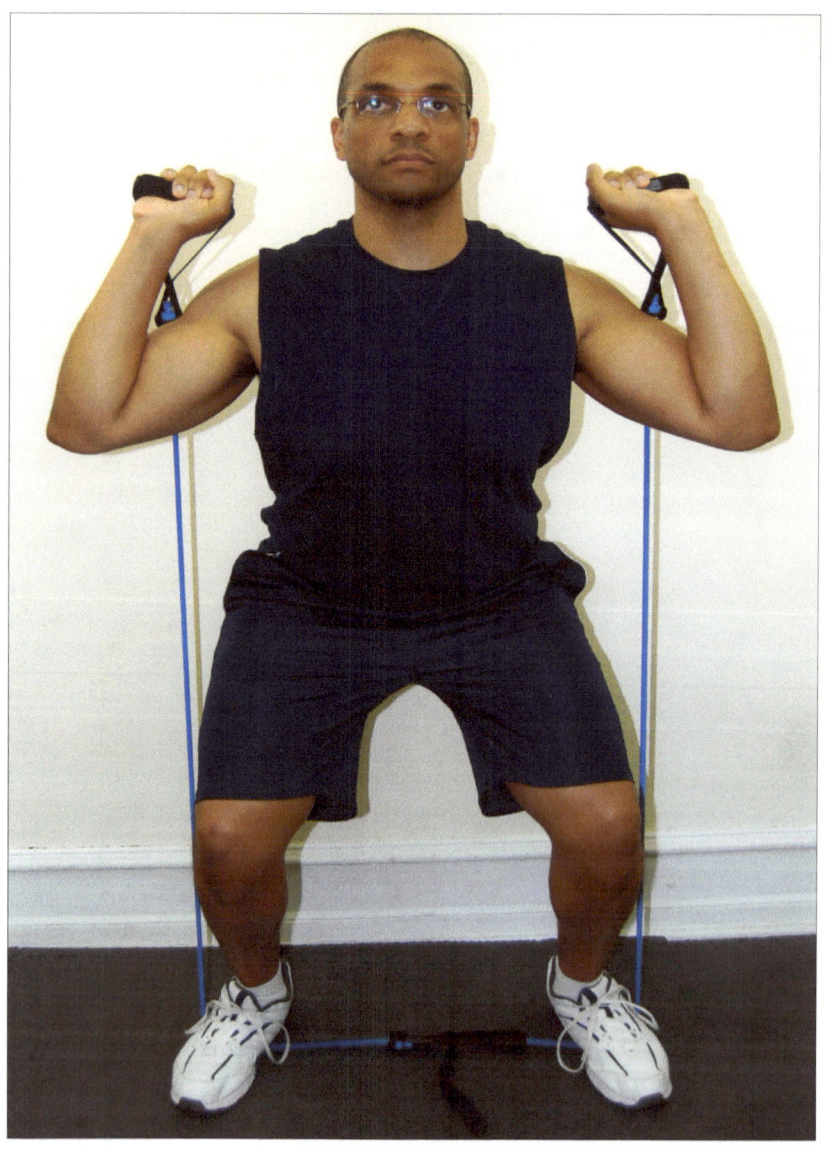

The exercises on the following pages will help to improve your overall movement during everyday activities. Keep in mind that all of the movements should only be performed following your doctor's approval to participate in physical activity. While performing the exercises, if you experience any pain or discomfort STOP the exercise and consult your physician.

STAYING ALIVE

The Staying Alive exercise targets the shoulders, core muscles, hips and thighs. Because this is a total body exercise, this exercise will also work your cardiovascular system. To perform this exercise, you will need to use an exercise band/tube or weights. Make sure that in the beginning, you perform this exercise with a low resistance or weight.

How to Perform the Exercise:

1. With your feet shoulder width apart, place the rubber tube/band under the arches of your feet with the handles crossed. One handle should be slightly longer than the other. The longer handle should be the working side and the shorter will serve your anchor.
2. Take hold of the longer handle with your right hand. Your right hand should be palm down and resting on your right thigh.
3. Facing forward, squat down so that your hips are almost level with your knees.
4. Begin to stand up, pushing through your heels.
5. As you are standing, raise your right hand from your right thigh, on a diagonal above your head.
6. After the first set is complete, switch hands and repeat steps 1-5.
7. Perform 3 sets of 10-15 repetitions.

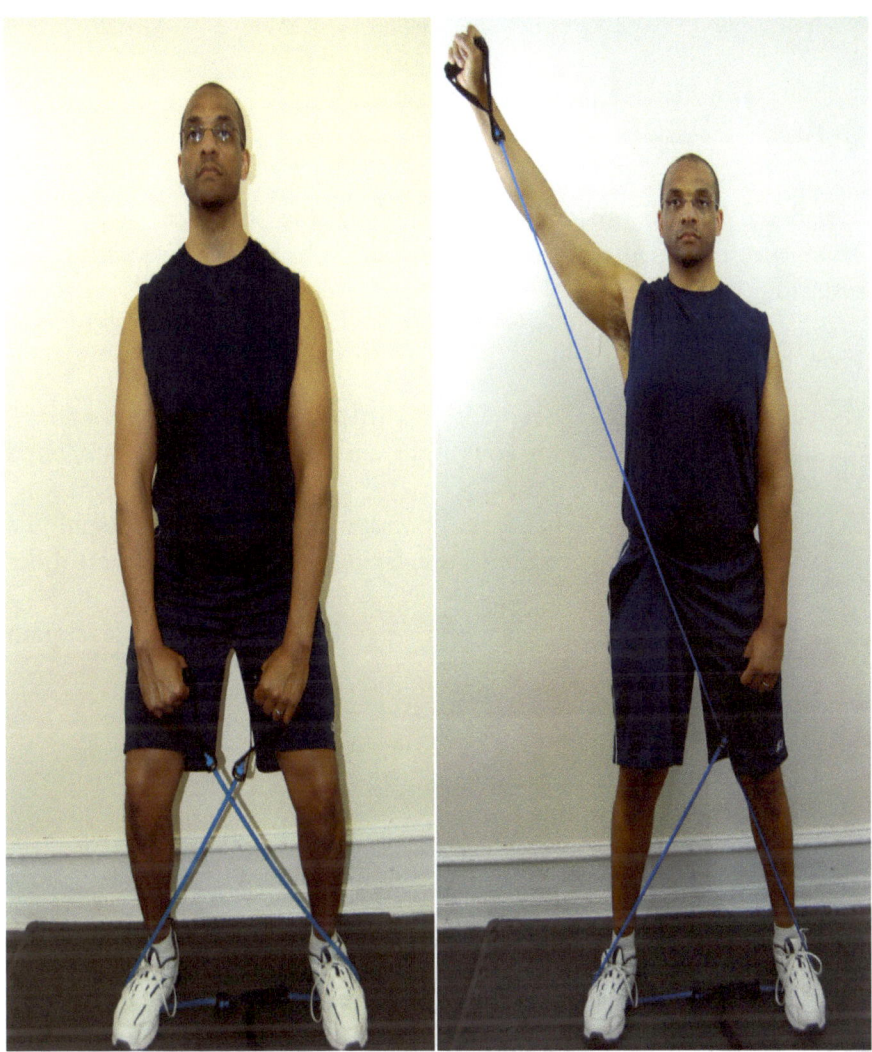

Start position   End position

SQUAT PRESS

The Squat Press is an exercise that targets the shoulders and thighs. Make sure that in the beginning, you perform this exercise with a low resistance or weight.

How to Perform the Exercise:

1. With your feet shoulder width apart, place the rubber tube/band under the arch of both your right and left foot. The tube/band should be equal in length.
2. Take hold of both handles. Bend your elbows and rotate the shoulders so that your palms are facing the ceiling and the rubber tubing/band is behind you.
3. Facing forward, squat down so that your hips are almost level with your knees.
4. Begin to stand up, pushing through your heels.
5. As you are standing, punch both hands up toward the ceiling.
6. Lower your hands and return to the starting position. Perform 3 sets of 10-15 repetitions.

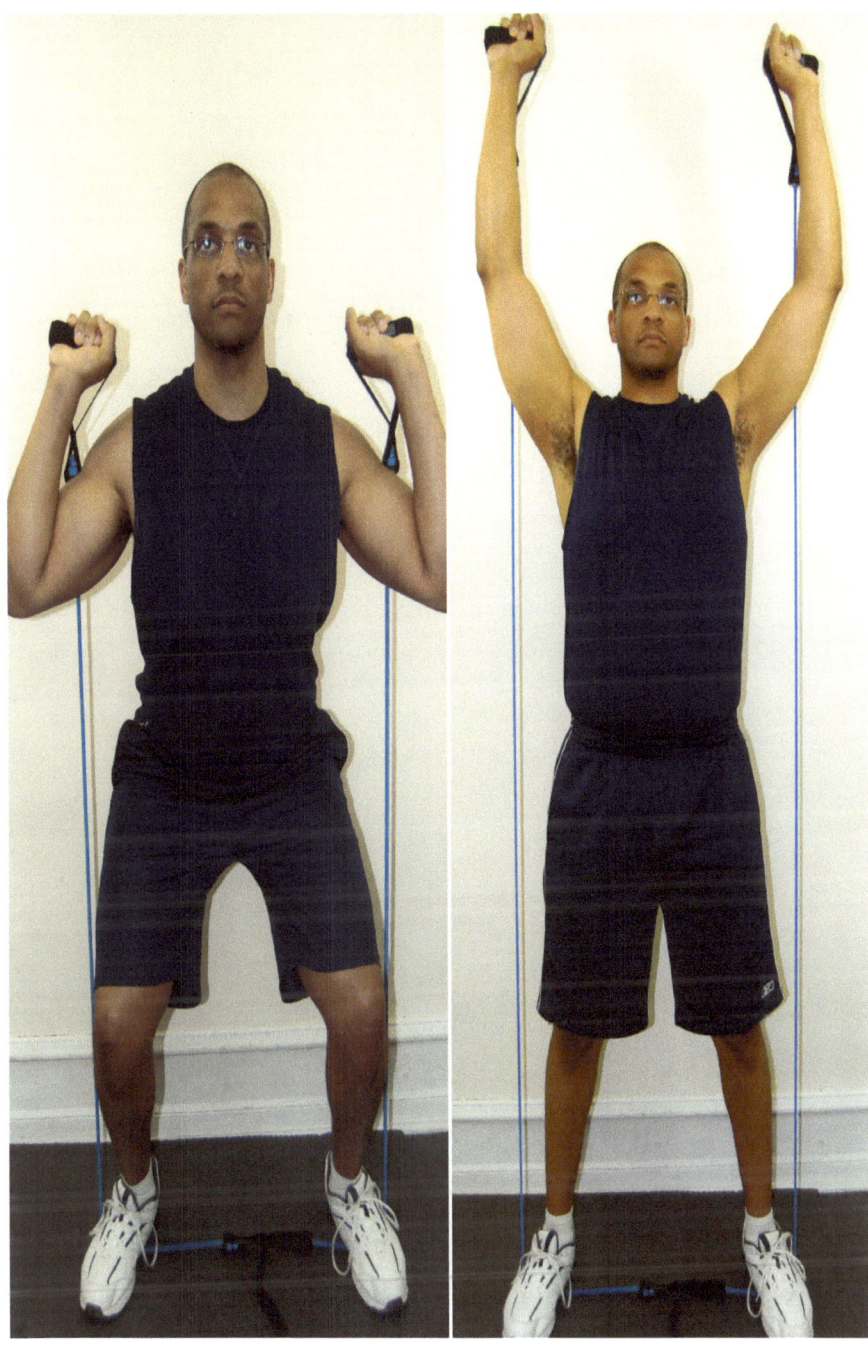

Start position   End position

SQUAT 'X'

This exercise is perfect for targeting every muscle of the body. This exercise is a variation on an Olympic lift that will be performed with the rubber tubes/bands. The exercise's primary targets are the shoulders, core muscles and thighs. Make sure that in the beginning, you perform this exercise with a low resistance or weight.

How to Perform the Exercise:

1. With your feet shoulder width apart, place the rubber tube/band under the arch of both your right and left foot. The tube/band should be equal in length.
2. Perform a handle exchange between the right and left hands so the tubing forms a "x" in front of you. Make sure you do not cross your hands; right hand should rest on your right thigh and your left hand should rest on your left thigh.
3. Facing forward, squat down so that your hips are almost level with your knees.
4. Stand up by pushing through your heels. Raise both hands off of your thighs and above your head.
5. Lower your hands and return to the starting position.
6. Perform 3 sets of 10-15 repetitions.

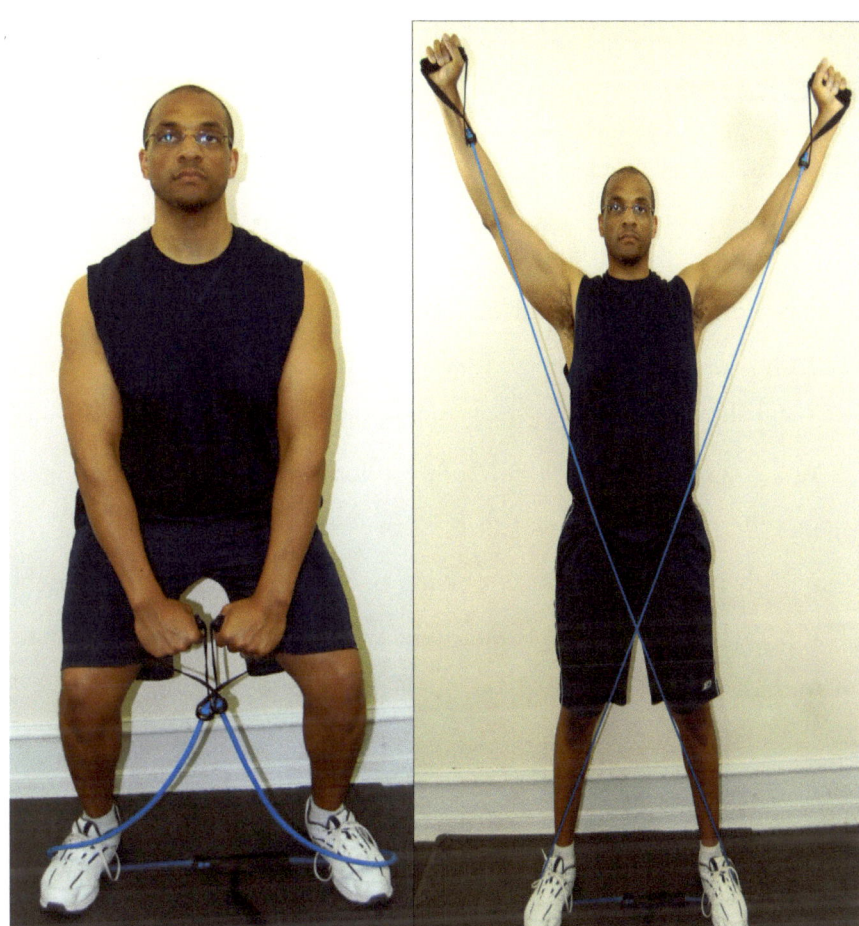

Start position   End position

SIDE RAISE

This exercise will work your shoulder muscles. Make sure that in the beginning, you perform this exercise with a low resistance or weight.

How to Perform the Exercise:

1. With your feet shoulder width apart, place the rubber band/tube under the arches of your feet, holding the band/tube in each hand. Make sure that the band/tube is long enough to reach your shoulders.

2. With hands resting on the outside of your thighs, raise your right arm out to the side, stopping when your hand is level with your shoulder. Left is at rest throughout the exercise.

3. Once at shoulder height, lower your right arm to the starting position.

4. Repeat on the left side.

5. Perform for 3 sets of 10-15 repetitions.

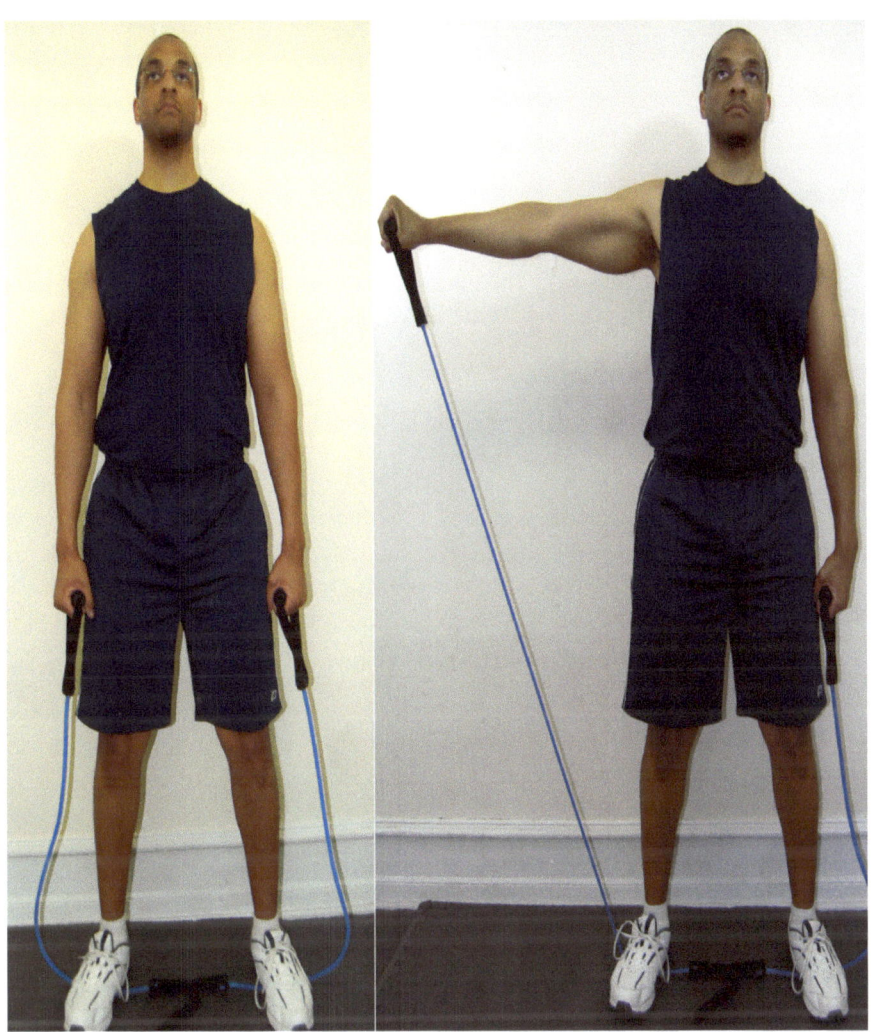

Start position   End position

FRONT RAISE

This exercise will work the muscles in front of your shoulders. Make sure that in the beginning, you perform this exercise with a low resistance or weight.

How to Perform the Exercise:

1. With your feet shoulder width apart, place the rubber band/tube under the arches of your feet. Make sure that the band/tube is long enough to reach your shoulders. Rest your hands on the front of your thighs.
2. Raise your right arm in front of you, stopping when your right hand is level with your right shoulder.
3. Once at shoulder height, lower your arm to the starting position.
4. Repeat with the left side.
5. Perform 3 sets of 10-15 repetitions.

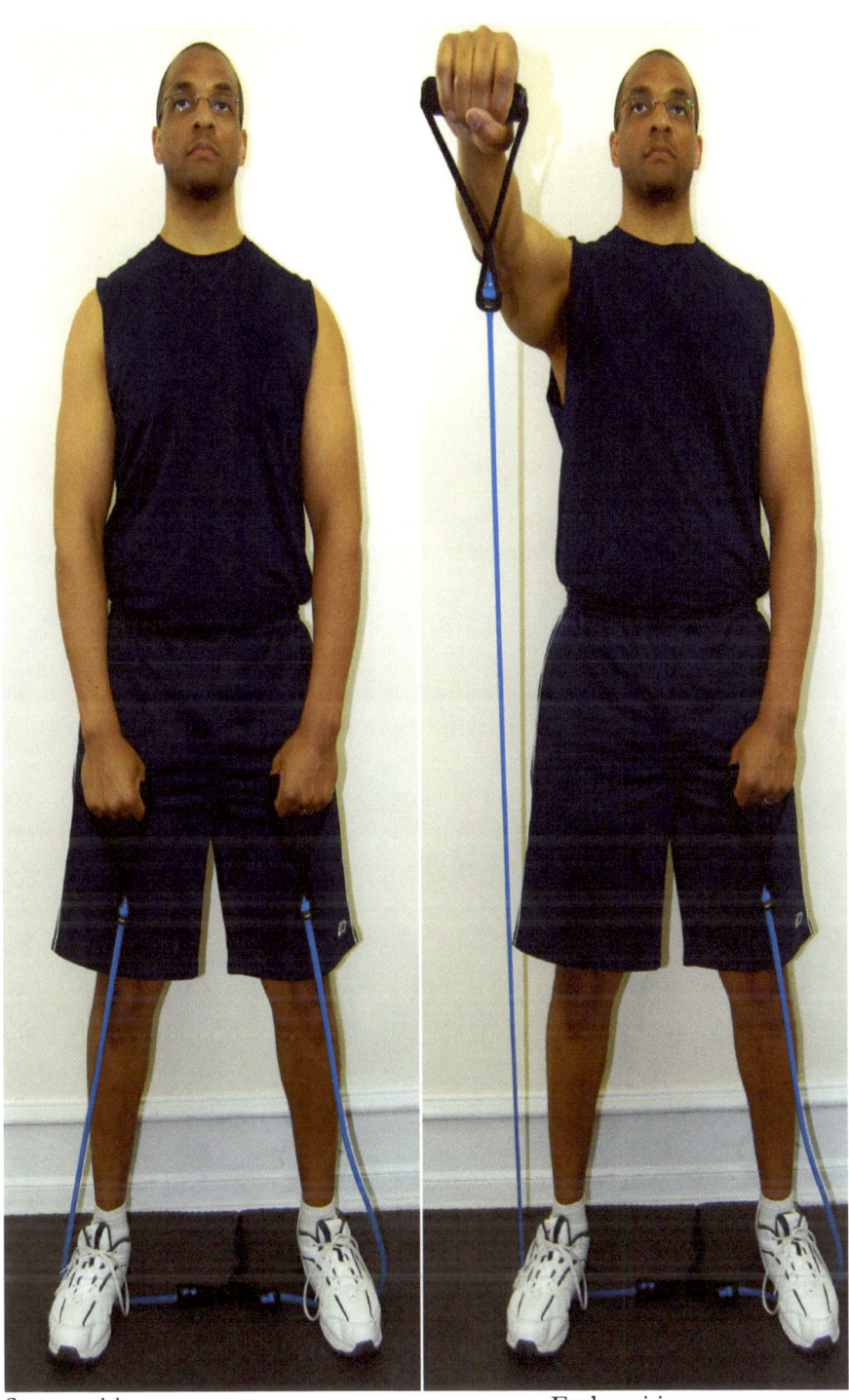

Start position   End position

SQUAT SIDE KICK (LEVEL 1)

This exercise will work the thighs and hip muscles. This exercise will also incorporate your cardiovascular system as well as work to improve your balance. Make sure that in the beginning, you perform this exercise with a low resistance or weight.

How to Perform the Exercise:

1. With your feet shoulder width apart, place the rubber band/tube under the arches of your feet. Take hold of both handles with your hands palm down and resting on your thighs.
2. Facing forward, squat down so that your hips are almost level with your knees.
3. As you are standing up, pushing through your heels, kick your right leg out to the side and lift your right foot up about 6 inches off of the ground.
4. Return your right foot to the starting position and squat again. As you are standing up, kick your left leg out to the side, lifting your left foot about 6 inches off of the ground.
5. Lower your left foot to the floor, returning to the starting position
6. Repeat for 2-3 sets of 10-15 repetitions.

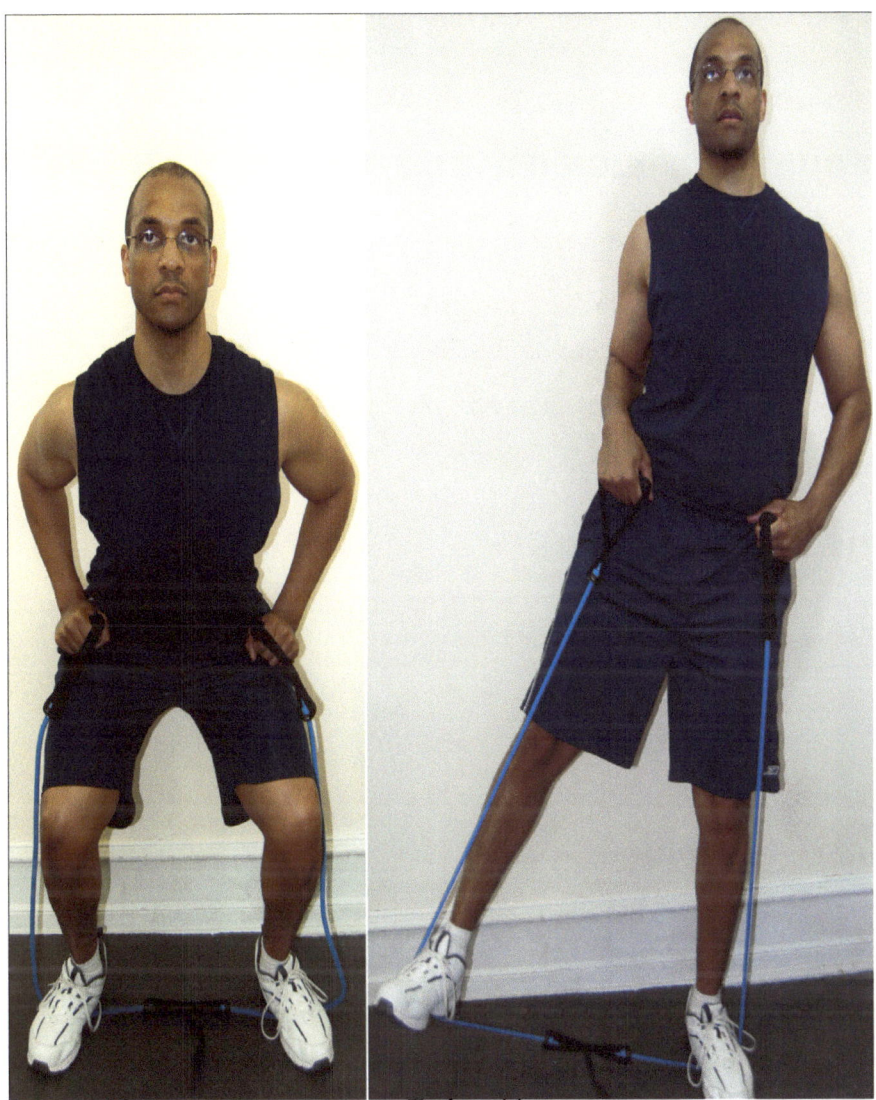

Start position   End position

SQUAT SIDE-KICK (LEVEL 2) WITH SIDE PUNCHES

This is an advanced version to the *Squat Side Kick* exercise. This exercise will work your shoulders, legs and hips, your balance as well as your cardiovascular system. Make sure that in the beginning, you perform this exercise with a low resistance or weight.

How to Perform the Exercise:

1. With your feet shoulder width apart, place the rubber band/tube under the arches of your feet. Cross your handles in front of you and take hold of both handles with your hands palm down and resting on your thighs.
2. Facing forward, squat down so that your hips are almost level with your knees.
3. As you are standing up, by pushing through your heels kicking your right leg out to the right side, while punching your left arm to the left side. This counts as 1 repetition.
4. Return to the starting position and squat again. This time, when standing up, kick your left leg out to the left side punching your right arm to the right side.
5. Repeat steps 1 through 4 for 2-3 sets of 10-15 repetitions.

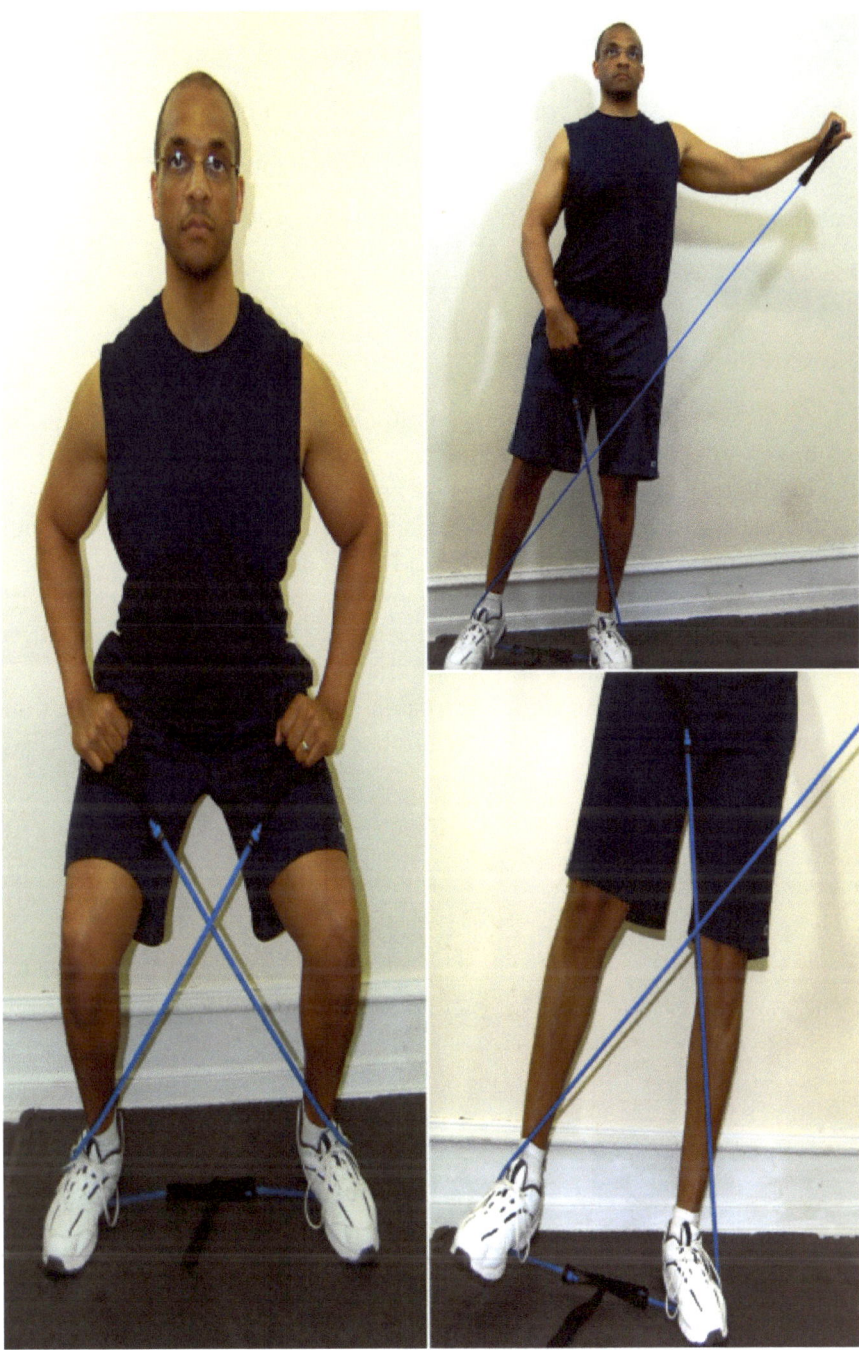

Start position   End position

CARDIO PUNCHES

This exercise will work your arms, chest, shoulders and cardiovascular system. This exercise may be performed with rubber tubes/bands, free weights or no weights at all. If using weights, start off with a light weight.

How to Perform the Exercise:

1. Stand with your feet shoulder width apart, with your knees slightly bent and your hands chest height.
2. Bend your elbows and bring your fists to shoulder height.
3. With or without weights in hands, begin to punch in front of you, one hand at a time, for a 15 second count.
4. Be sure to alternate hands and perform as many as you can in 15 seconds. Make sure that the non-working hand stays in an elevated position (elbow height and fist by the shoulder).
5. Perform 2 to 3 sets, only increasing the amount of time that you punch by 5 seconds as the exercise becomes easier.

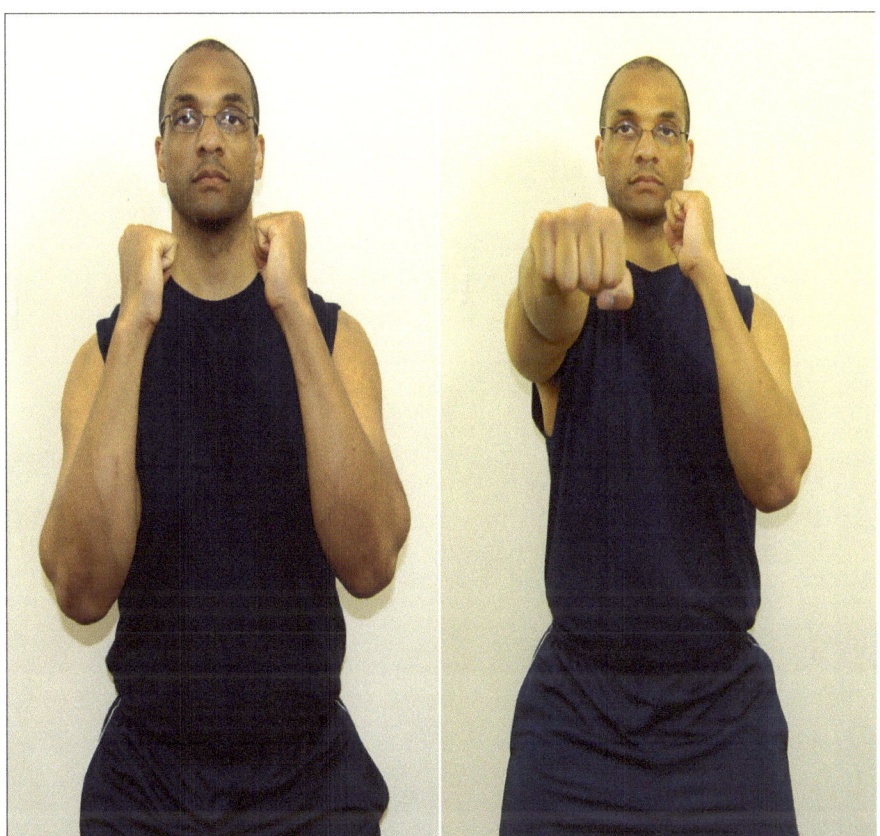

Start position   End position

KICK-BACKS (LEVEL 1)

This exercise will target the gluteal muscles along with your abdominal muscles and your balance. Make sure that in the beginning, you perform this exercise with a low resistance or weight.

How to Perform the Exercise:

1. Start this exercise on your hands and knees. Make sure that you have placed a mat on the floor to protect your hands and knees.
2. Place the rubber band/tube around the arch of your right foot, holding a handle in each hand.
3. Holding on to the band/tube, kick your right foot straight behind you, extending your right leg.
4. Repeat for 10-15 repetitions for 2-3 sets.
5. Following the final set, switch the band/tube to your left foot.

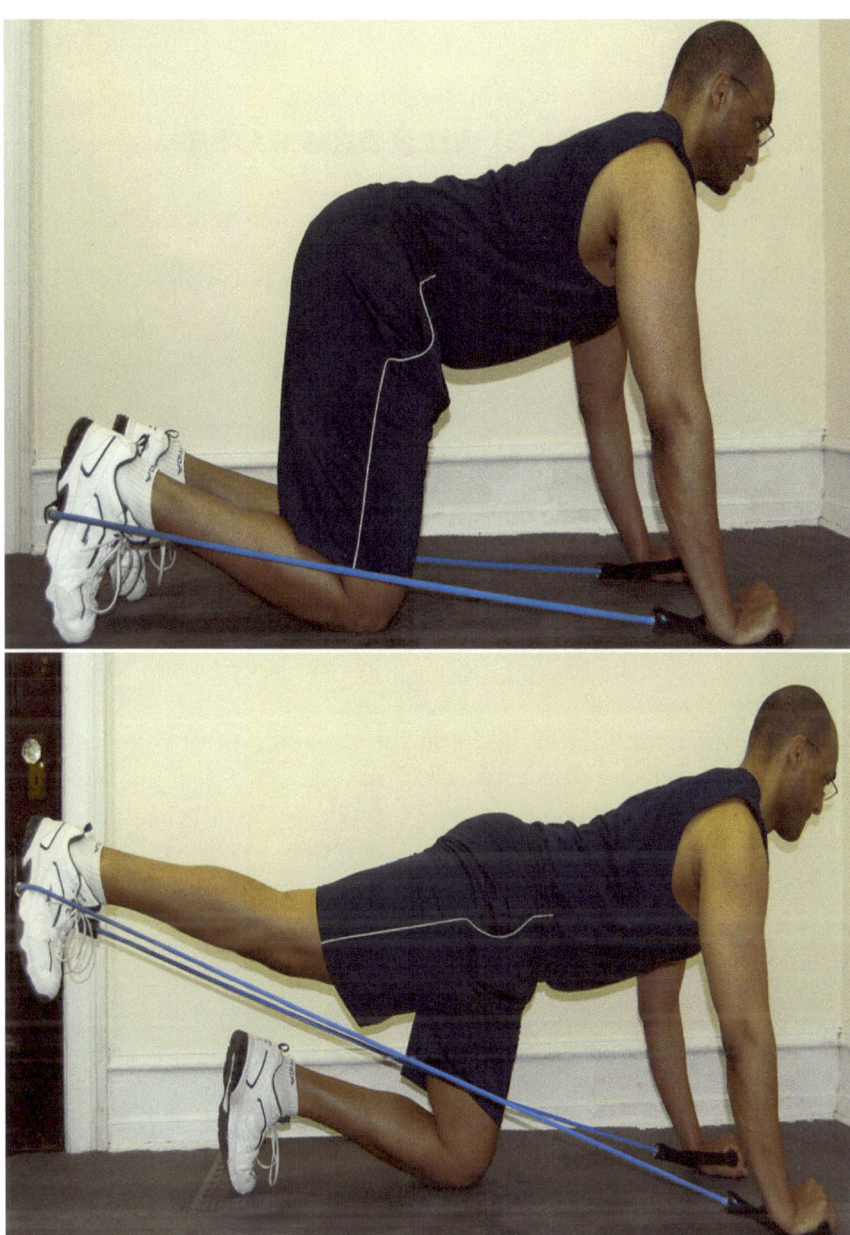

Top picture: Start position   Bottom picture: End position

KICK-BACK (LEVEL 2) WITH ARM RAISE

This is an advanced exercise to the traditional kick-back that will target the gluteal and abdominal muscles. This exercise will also work your balance. Make sure that in the beginning, you perform this exercise with a low resistance or weight.

How to Perform the Exercise:

1. Start this exercise on your hands and knees. Make sure that you have placed a mat on the floor to protect your hands and knees.
2. Place the rubber band/tube around the arch of your right foot, holding a handle in each hand.
3. Holding on to the band/tube, suck in your belly button to prevent arching of the back.
4. Kick your right foot behind you by extending both your right leg AND your left arm to shoulder height.
5. Repeat for 10-15 repetitions for 2-3 sets.
6. Following the final set, switch the band/tube to your left foot.

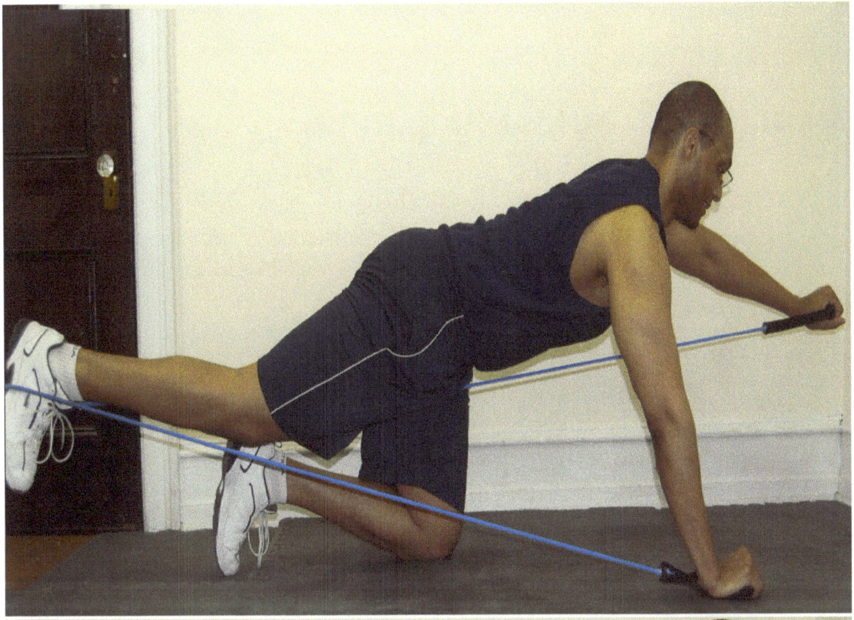

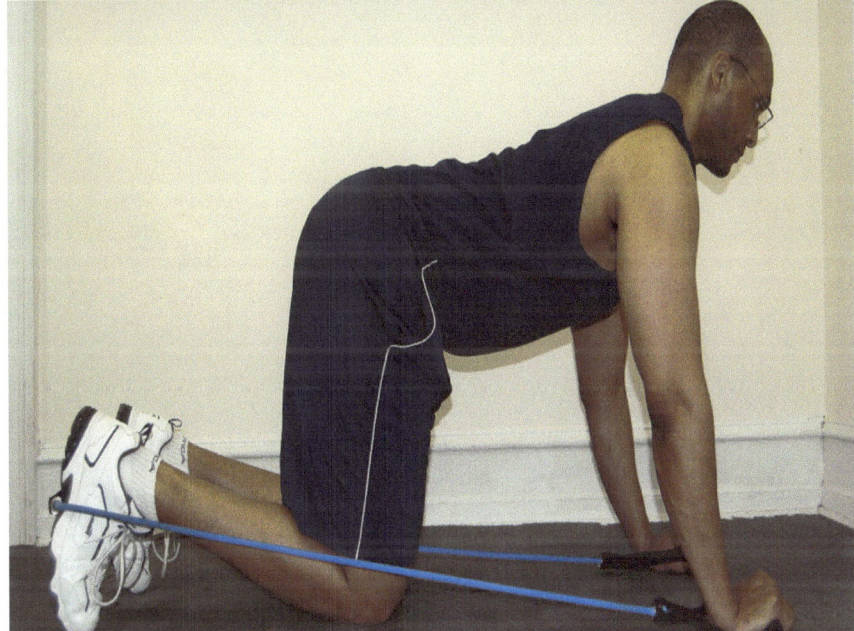

Top picture: End position   Bottom picture: Start position

TRADITIONAL PUSH-UPS (LEVEL 1)

This exercise will work your chest, shoulder and abdominal muscles. This is a *Level 1* exercise because it is performed on your knees.

How to Perform the Exercise:

1. Lie on your stomach with your hands under your shoulders and your feet shoulder width apart.
2. Suck in your belly button to help keep your back straight.
3. Keeping your knees on the and while keeping your body straight (parallel to the floor), push your body off the floor until your arms are almost straight.
4. After rising to the top of the push-up, slowly lower yourself toward the floor, stopping when your elbows are level with your chest. Your elbows will be at a 90-degree angle.
5. Repeat for 10 repetitions for 2-3 sets.

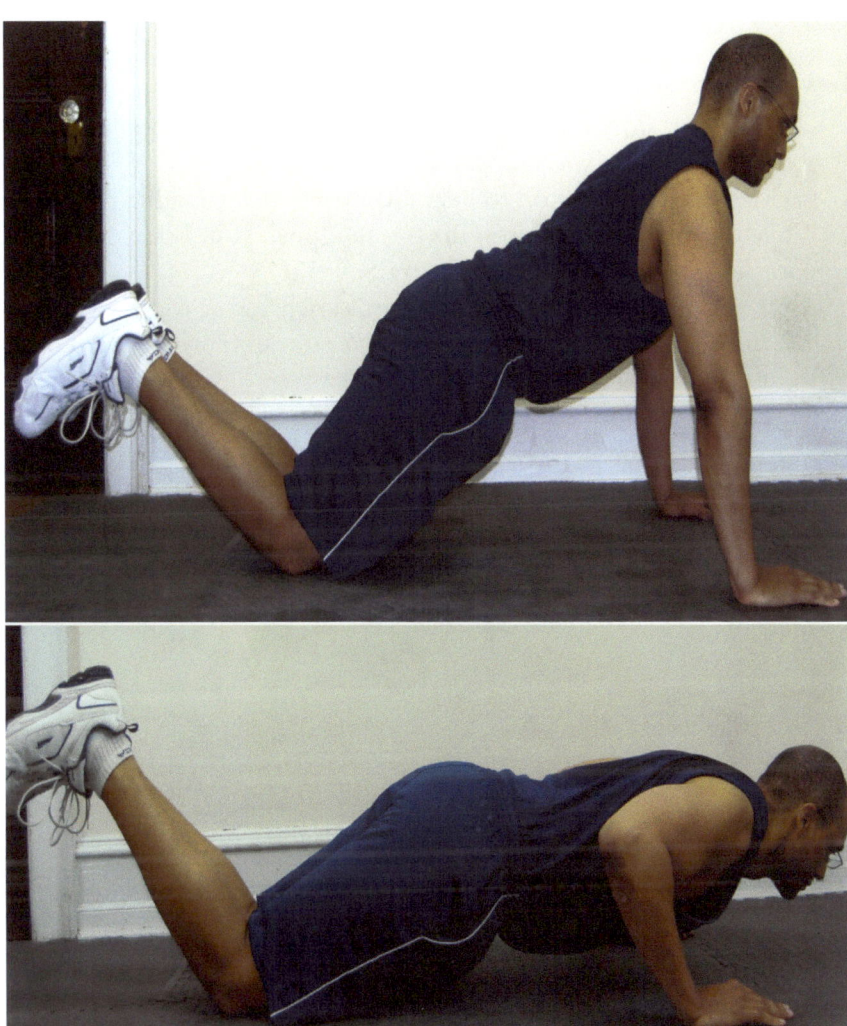

Top picture: Start position   Bottom picture: End position

TRADITIONAL PUSH-UPS (LEVEL 2)

This exercise is a natural progression of the Level 1 push-up, which will further work the chest, shoulder and abdominal muscles.

How to Perform the Exercise:

1. Lie on your stomach with your hands under your shoulders and your feet shoulder width apart.
2. Suck in your belly button to help keep your back straight.
3. While digging your toes into the ground, push your body off of the floor until your arms are almost straight.
4. After rising to the top of the push-up, slowly lower yourself toward the floor, stopping when your elbows are level with your chest. Your elbows will be at a 90-degree angle.
5. Repeat 10 repetitions for 2-3 sets.

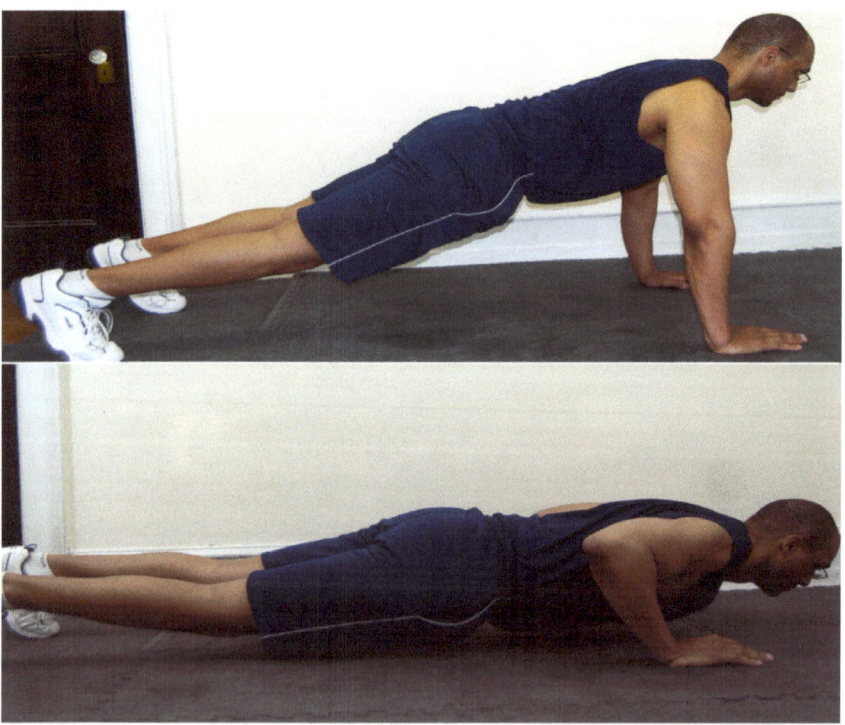

Top picture: Start position   Bottom picture: End position

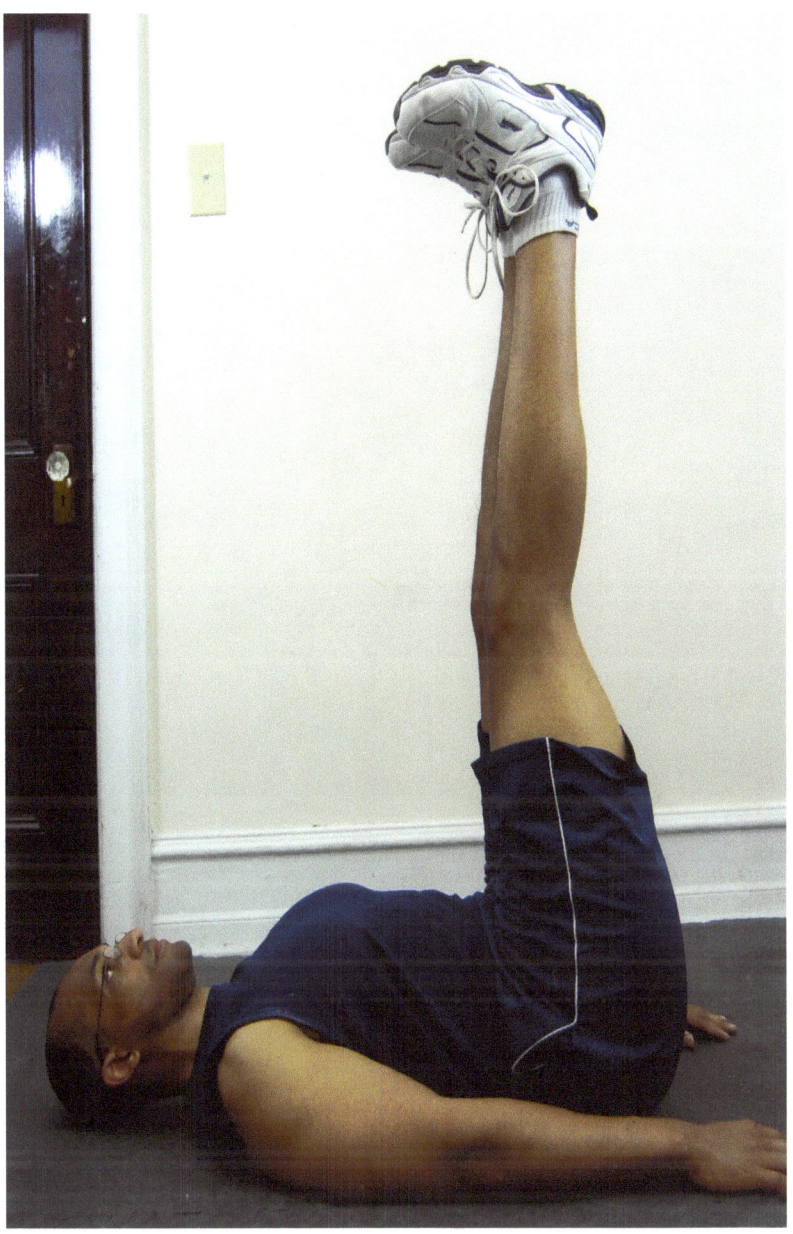

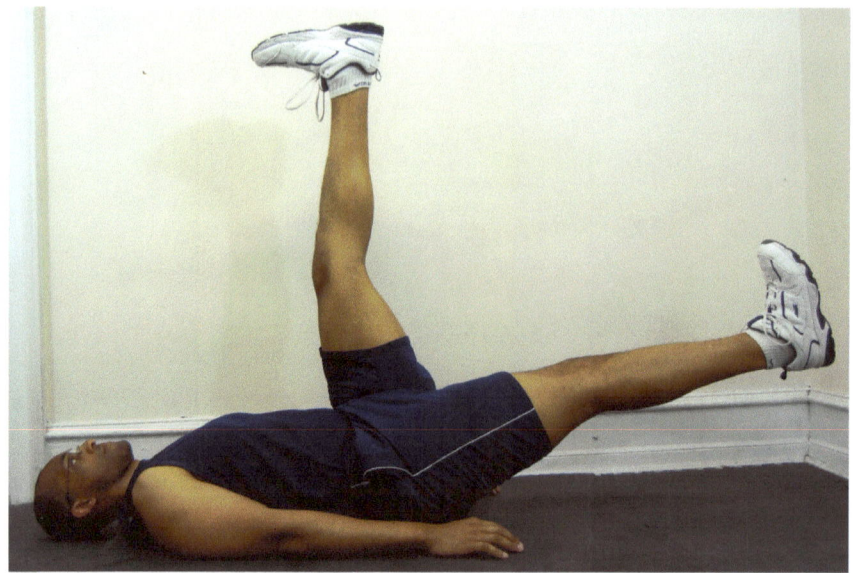

Performing Scissor Kick

SLOW SCISSOR KICK

This exercise targets the abdominal muscles as well as the muscles of the upper thigh.

How to Perform the Exercise:

1. Lie down on the floor on your back. **Make sure that your back is *flat* on the floor.** Raise your legs so that they are perpendicular to the floor and the soles of your feet are facing the ceiling. *Alternate position:* With your knees bent, lift your knees so that your feet are off of the floor.
2. Suck in your belly button to keep the back straight without arching your back, slowly begin to lower your right leg toward the floor while keeping your left leg straight in the air. Stop lowering your right leg when you get about an inch off of the floor. *Alternate position:* Your knees bent, lower your right leg until your right foot touches the floor. Bring your right leg back up until it's parallel to the left leg.
3. Now switch legs, leaving your right leg in the starting position and lower the left leg to the floor.
4. Repeat for 2-3 sets of 10 repetitions.

Dr. Brian K. Walls

MOVEMENT 4: TESTING YOUR ABILITY TO MOVE

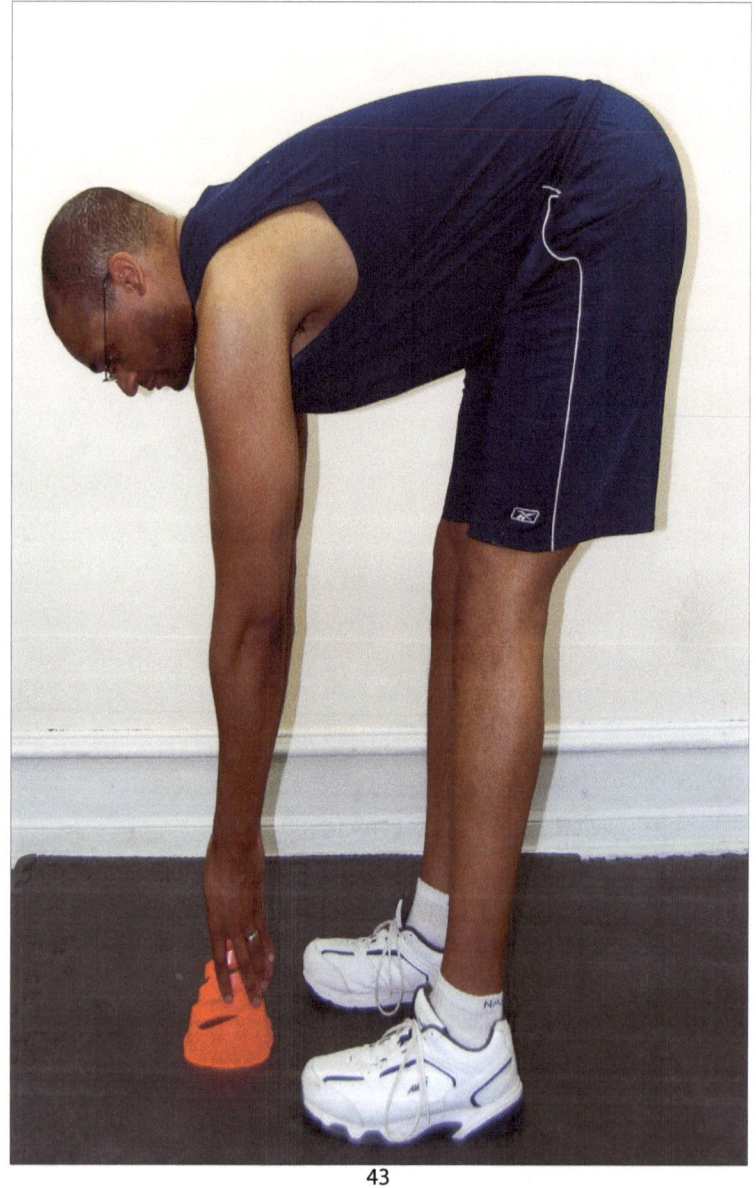

The following pages offer a few physical tests that will allow you to grade yourself using the score sheet below to assess how easily you can perform your everyday movements. When scoring, if you are unsure of the score to give yourself, give yourself the lower score. As you keep exercising, your score will improve over time.

Movement Score Sheet

Name: Age:	Date:	Date:
Sit to Stand		
Pick Up Object		
Push-up		

When performing the physical tests be sure that there is supervision available to protect against possible injury.

What are Compensations? According to Webster's dictionary, compensation is a defect or loss of an organ by increased functioning of another unimpaired organ. For our purposes, compensation is the body's ability to perform a movement by using the stronger body part to perform a motion. By doing so, the side of the body that is "going along for the ride", becomes weaker, which creates a muscle imbalance within the body. This muscle imbalance may then lead to injuries within the body.

SIT-TO-STAND

Sit-to-stand is a test that will reveal how well you are able to stand from a seated position. In addition to testing your ability to stand from a chair, this test will also reveal the strength of both your legs and stomach muscles because it is done without the use of your hands. I have altered the normal standing motion by asking you to place your hands behind your head, which forces you to utilize your leg and stomach muscles. The placement of your arms behind your head also allows you to assess how tight your chest and shoulder muscles may be.

Starting position: Using a chair with arm rests that is 35 or 36 inches in height, sit on the front of the chair with your feet flat on the floor and shoulder width. Relax your shoulders and place your hands behind your head. If you are unable to place your hands behind your head, cross your arms over your chest.

Movement: Take a deep breath, engaging your stomach muscles. Press your feet into the floor, pushing through your mid-foot and heel, until you are standing tall with your hands remaining behind your head.

Possible compensations include placing one foot in front of the other, placing body weight on one leg to rise out of the chair, using the arm rest to stand up from the chair, or using an assistive device in addition to the arm rest to get out of the chair.

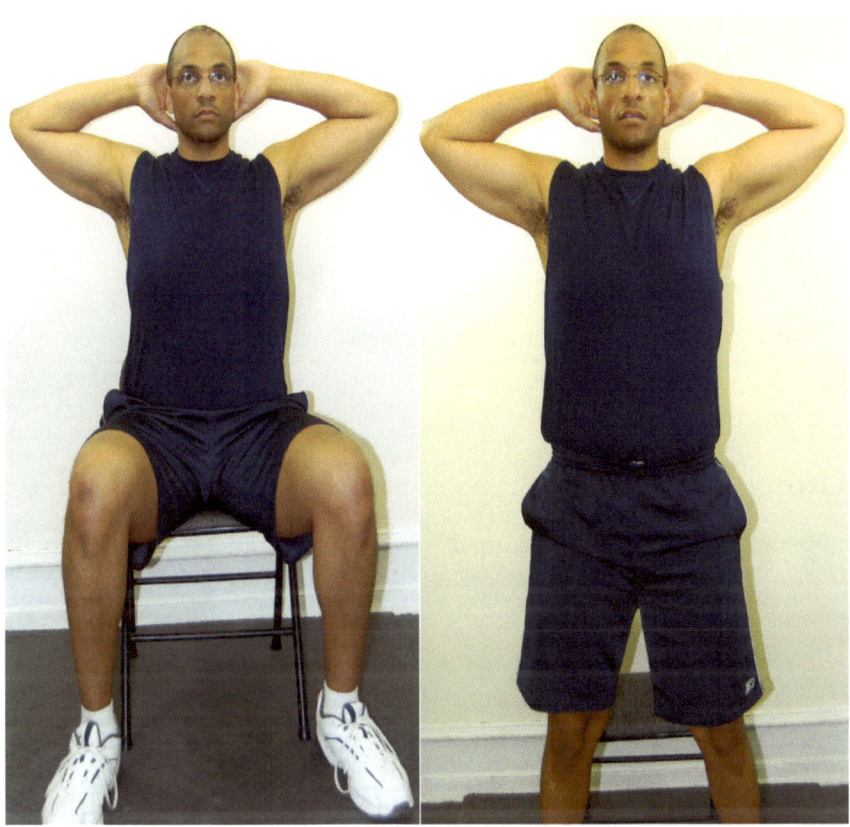

Start position   End position

Scoring:

Score of Zero (0): Unable to complete movement.

Score of One (1): Able to complete movement with assistance of arm rest and compensations.

Score of Two (2): Able to complete movement with assistance of arm rest.

Score of Three (3): Able to complete movement without any *compensations*.

PICK UP OBJECT

Pick Up Object test determines the flexibility in your lower back and legs. This test mimics a motion that is performed numerous times throughout the day. The first time you perform this movement, you may **not** give yourself a high score. That is all right! As long as you are performing the stretches from Movement #2 in this book, you will improve your score on this test.

Starting Position: Stand with your arms on the side of your body and your legs straight, approximately 3 inches behind a 6-inch object.

Movement: Keeping your legs straight, slowly bend forward reaching out with your arms to pick up the object with your legs still straight. Grab the object with both hands and return to the starting position.

Possible compensations include leaning on one leg to pick up the object, also known as the "Golfers" technique. This movement may be done using the back of a chair to pick up the object or bending your knees to squat down to pick up the object. Another possible compensation is having someone hold your waist while performing the movement.

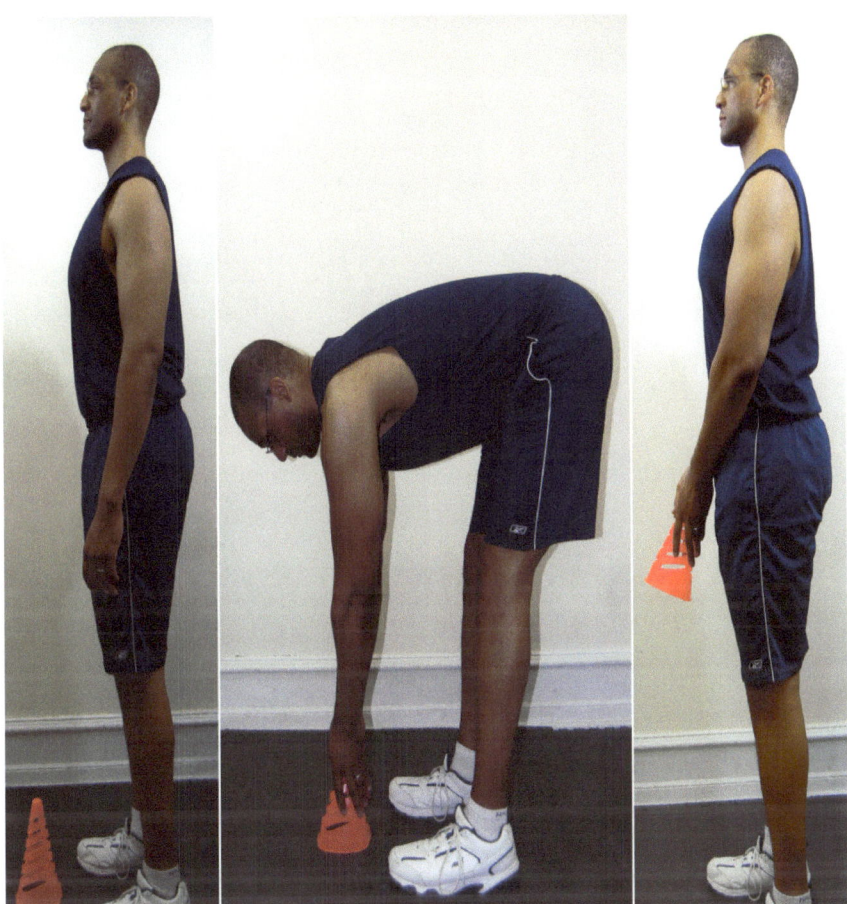

Start position   End position

Scoring:

Score of Zero (0): Pain, unable to perform movement.

Score of One (1): Able to perform movement with body supported.

Score of Two (2): Able to perform movement with compensations.

Score of Three (3): Able to perform movement *without any compensations*.

PUSH-UPS

Push-ups tests your upper-body strength. Most people ask why it's important to perform a push-up. The push-up is a movement that we do every day we get up from bed. Perhaps you are not in the traditional push-up position, but I assure you that you are pushing yourself up which requires upper body strength in your chest, shoulders and abdominal muscles. The ability to perform push-ups is a quick and easy self-test on how well you are moving, and is one you can use throughout your lifetime.

Starting Position: Using a mat, lying face down on the floor, with your feet/knees at shoulder width and your hands under your shoulders.

Movement: Keeping your body in a straight line, take a breath and push through your hands, stopping when you have almost reached full elbow extension. Do not lock your elbows straight! Count the number of push-ups you are able to perform in 60 seconds.

Possible Compensations include allowing your hips to drop or pushing your hips up in the air. Other compensations include the alternative methods described below:

Alternative Push-Ups:

Wall Push-ups:
1. Stand arms' length from a wall, placing your hands on the wall at shoulder width and shoulder height. Your heels should be slightly off of the floor.
2. Keeping your body straight, suck in your belly button and bending your elbows, lower yourself toward the wall. Stop when your elbows are level with your chest.
3. Push out against the wall, returning to the starting position.

Chair Push-Ups:
1. Place a chair against a wall with the back of the chair on the wall. Place your hands on either side of the chair's seat in the push-up position. Your heels should be off of the floor.
2. Keeping your body straight, suck in your belly button and lower yourself toward the chair. Stop when your elbows are level with your chest.
3. Push against the chair, returning to the starting position.

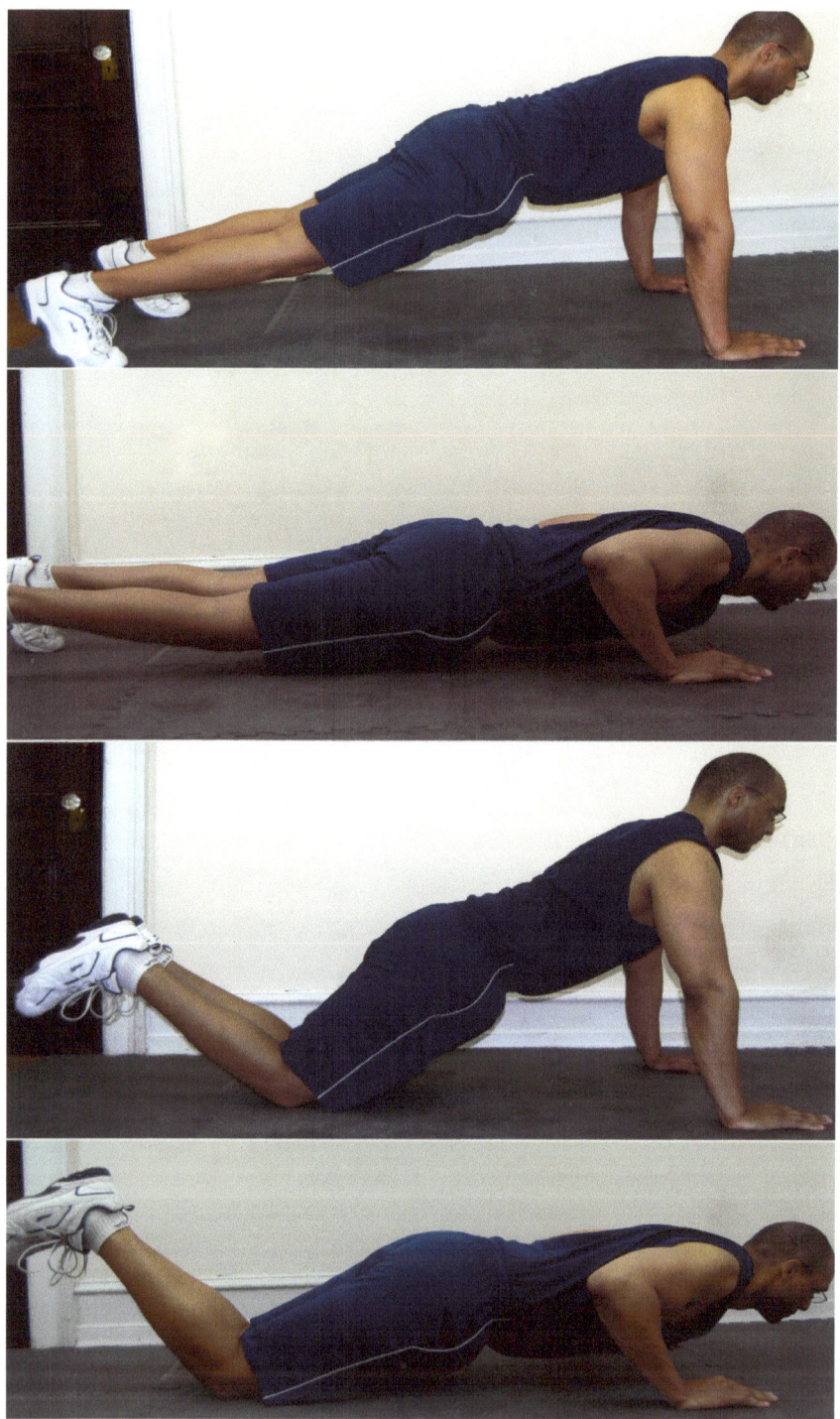

Scoring:

Score of Zero (0): Pain

Score of Zero (1): Performed push-up on the wall.

Score of Zero (2): Performed push-up on a chair.

Score of Zero (3): Able to perform movement.

SAMPLE WORKOUT ROUTINE

Working out does not have to take 60 minutes. The adage "quality over quantity" also holds true with respect to exercise. The beauty of the exercises shown in this book is that the majority of them work the entire body and eventually will shorten the amount of time that is required. Those exercises also may be used as a supplement to your established workout program "quick" 10-15 minute program that will strengthen the muscular and cardiovascular systems.

Here is an example of a "quick" workout:

1.   Cardio Punches: 3 sets of 10 seconds (p. 28)

2.   Squat X: 2 sets of 10 repetitions (p.18)

3.   Squat Press: 2 sets of 10 repetitions (p. 16)

4.   Front Raise: 2 sets of 10 repetitions (p. 22)

5.   Kick-Backs (Level 1): 2 sets of 10 repetitions (p. 30)

6.   Push-Ups (Level 1): 2 sets of 10 repetitions (p. 34)

7.   Cardio Punches: 3 sets of 15 seconds (p. 28)

When performing the "quick" workout routine, take a 15-30 second break between each set and each exercise. By working out with short breaks, you will work your cardiovascular system along with your muscles. As always, if you are experiencing any discomfort while performing the exercises, STOP the exercise.

REFERENCES

1. Berg, K. and Norman, K. (1996). Functional Assessment of Balance and Gait. *Clinics of Geriatric Medicine 12*:705.
2. Burton, L. & Cook, E.G. (2004). *Athletic Body in Balance; Optimal Movement Skills and Conditioning for Performance.* Champaign, IL: Human Kinetics.
3. Tinetti, M. (1986). Performance-oriented assessment of mobility problems in elderly patients. *Journal of American Geriatrics Society 34*:119.

RESPONSES ABOUT *EXERCISE FOR THE ATHLETE WITHIN:*

"Read it. Loved it! Love how basic and to the point it is. The average person can pick it up and read it and commit to it!"
- Donna Storm, Fitness Expert and Radio Personality

"The straightforward illustrations and instructions ensure correct form and explain which muscles are being used. I highly recommend this book as an excellent guide to improve everyday movement."
- Elise Lamarra, Vice President of Clinical Operations, Friends Life Care

ABOUT THE AUTHOR

Dr. Brian Walls, USAW, AAAI is the Director of Strength and Conditioning for Whole Health 4 You a fitness and rehabilitation company located in Philadelphia, PA. He has assisted numerous individuals in improving their movement within their daily lives both on and off the athletic playing field.